Evan the Vegan Boy

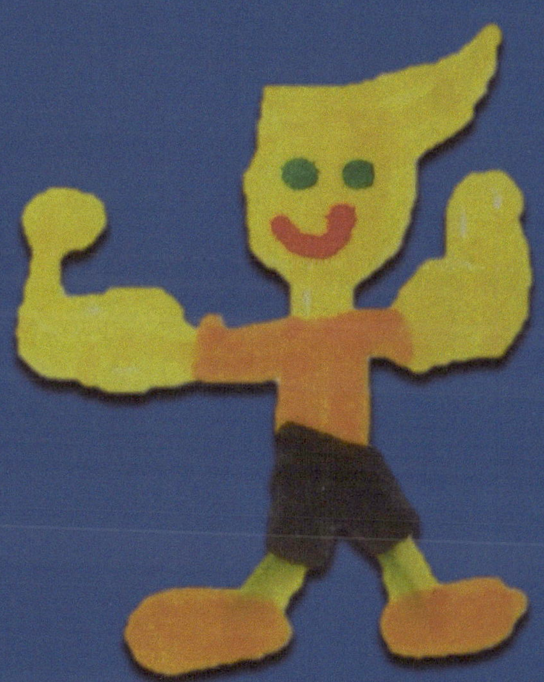

Evan the Vegan Boy

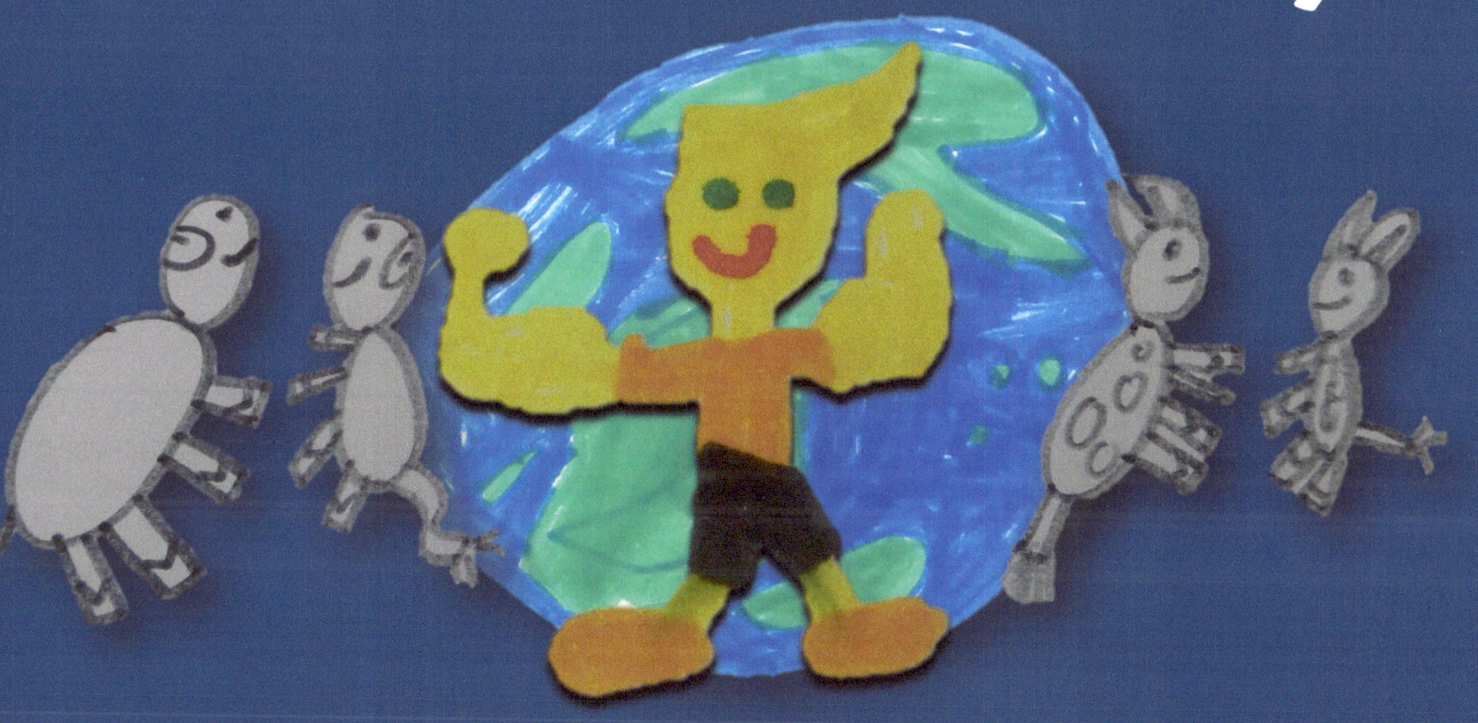

Written by Andy and Laura Greger

Illustrated by Violet and Evan Greger

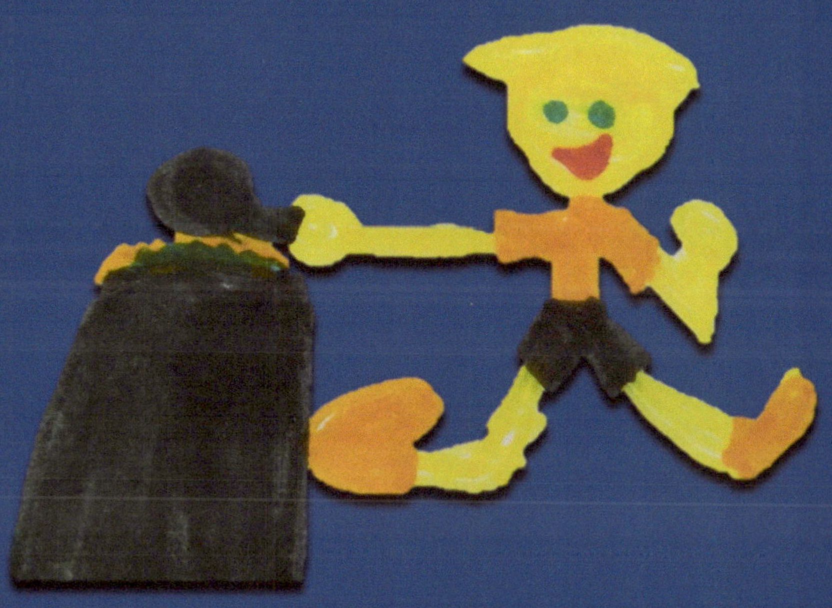

They call me little chef, but my name is really Evan.

I may be five and a half, but I cook like I'm eleven.

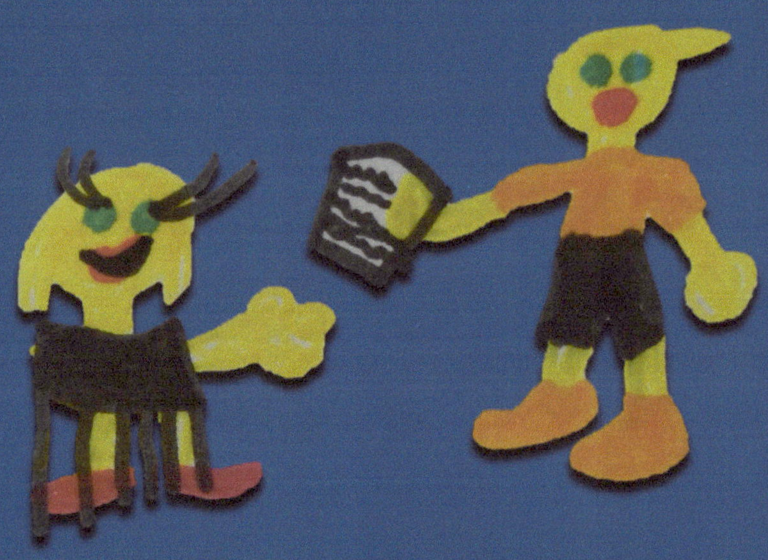

The things I like to cook are vegan through and through.

And if you'd like to stick around, I'll make you something new.

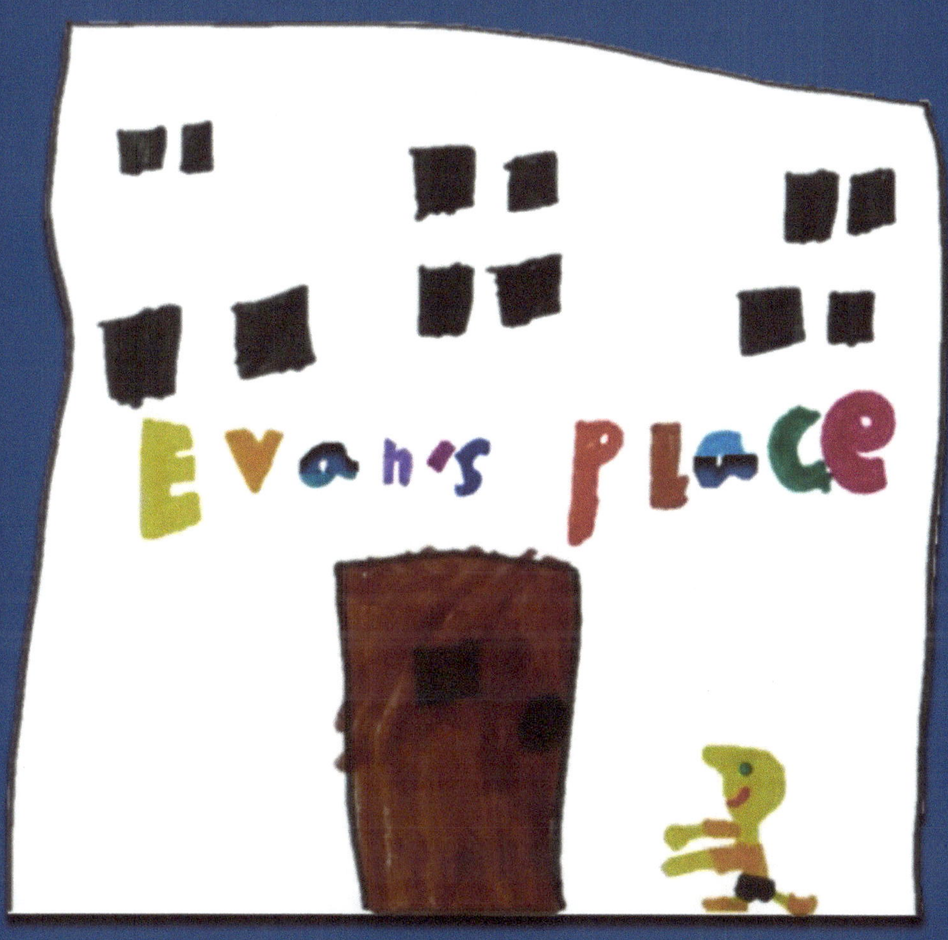

Get ready for a bunch of meals, with food I love to eat.

Maybe one day I'll own a restaurant, where you can take a seat.

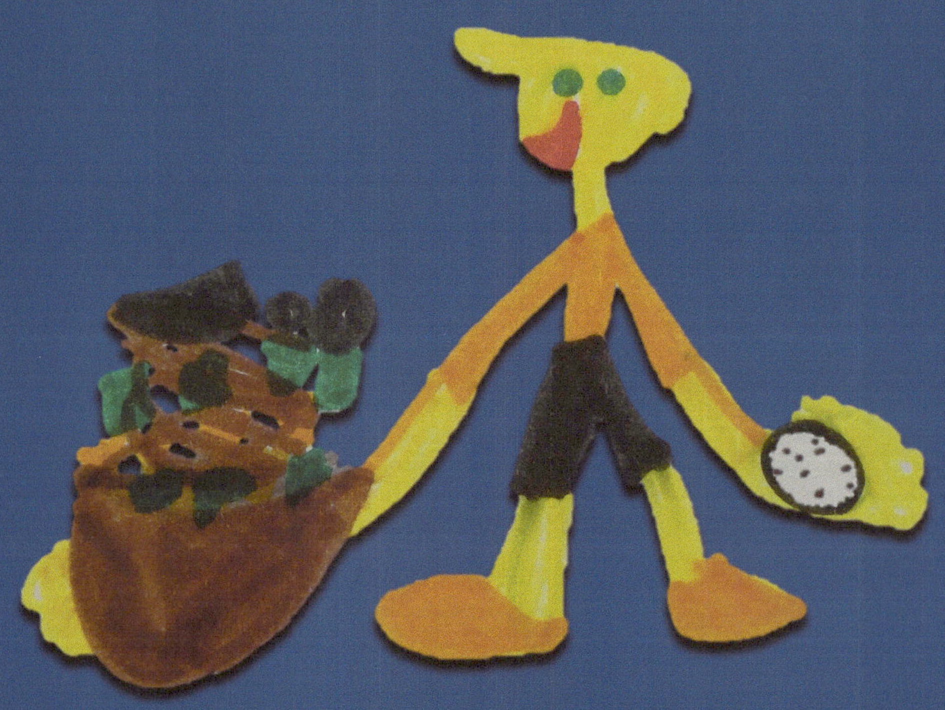

One of my favorite meals is called a sushi bowl.

There's cucumbers, rice, and carrots; sometimes it's in a roll.

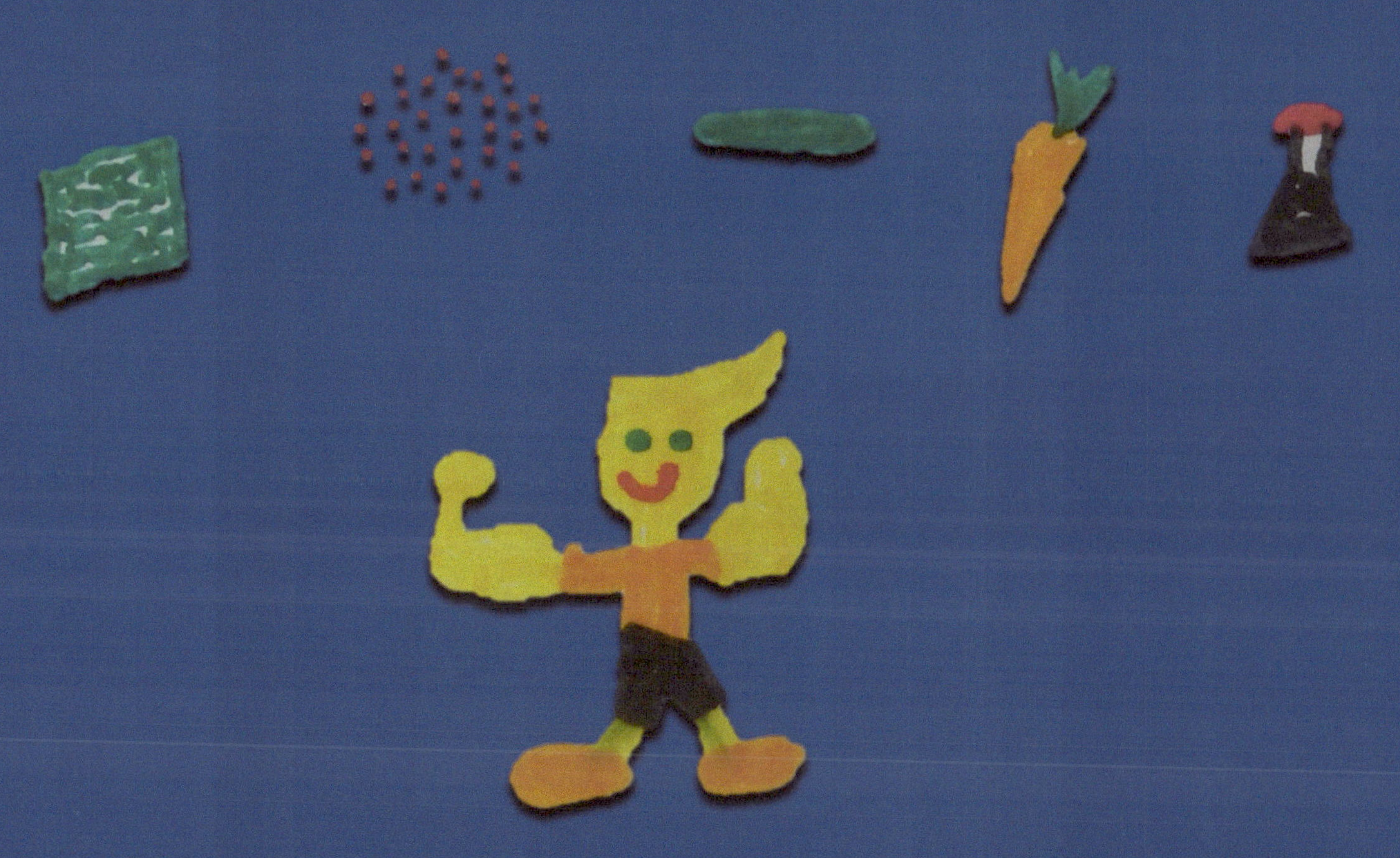

I usually add some soy sauce and a little roasted seaweed.

I feel so big and strong because it has all the protein I need.

Pizza Oven

Next is a tasty pizza, I whip it up with ease.

It's like a veggie lover, just subtract the cheese.

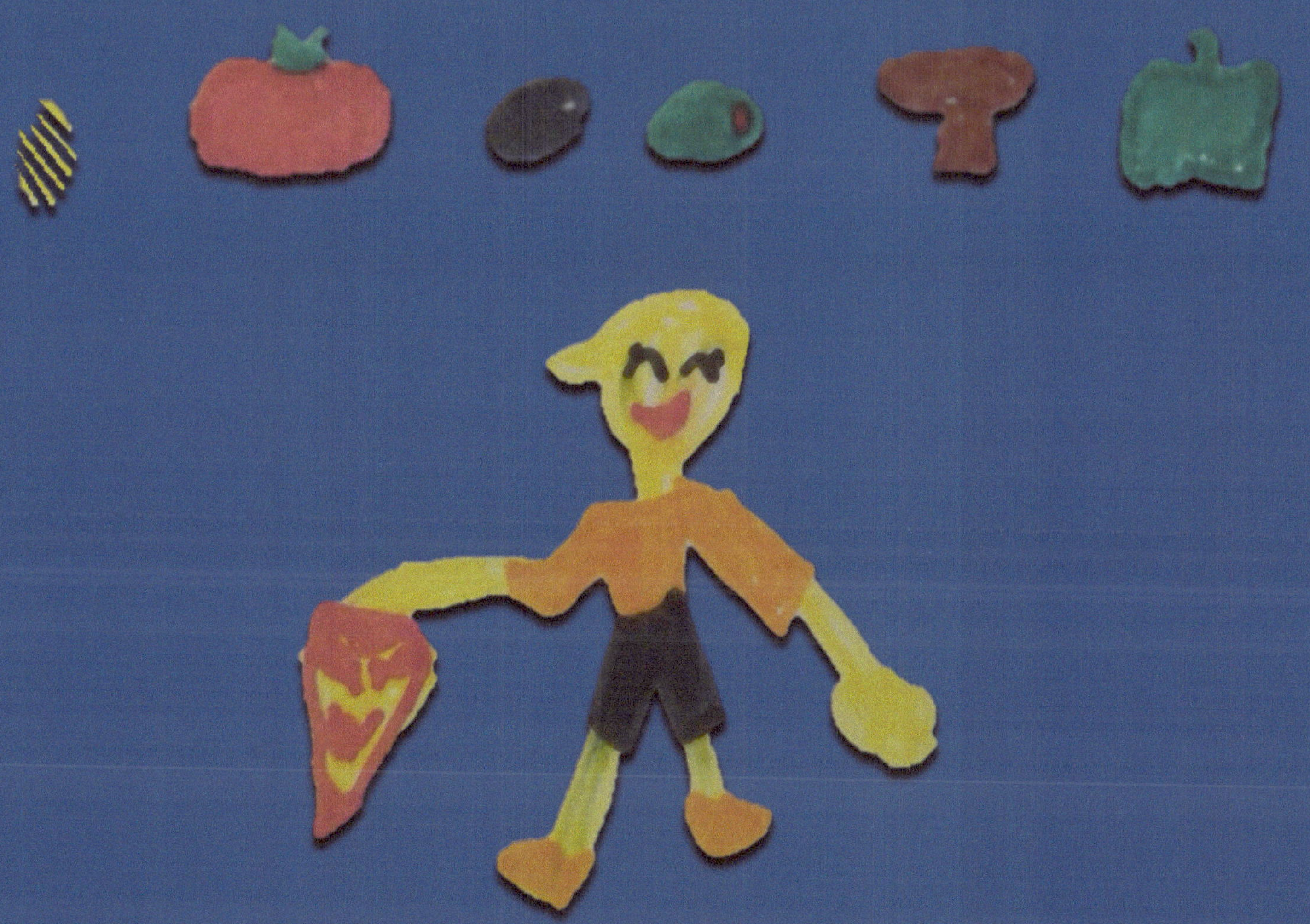

You could add vegan cheese, a lot or just a pinch.

I prefer sauce and veggies covering every inch.

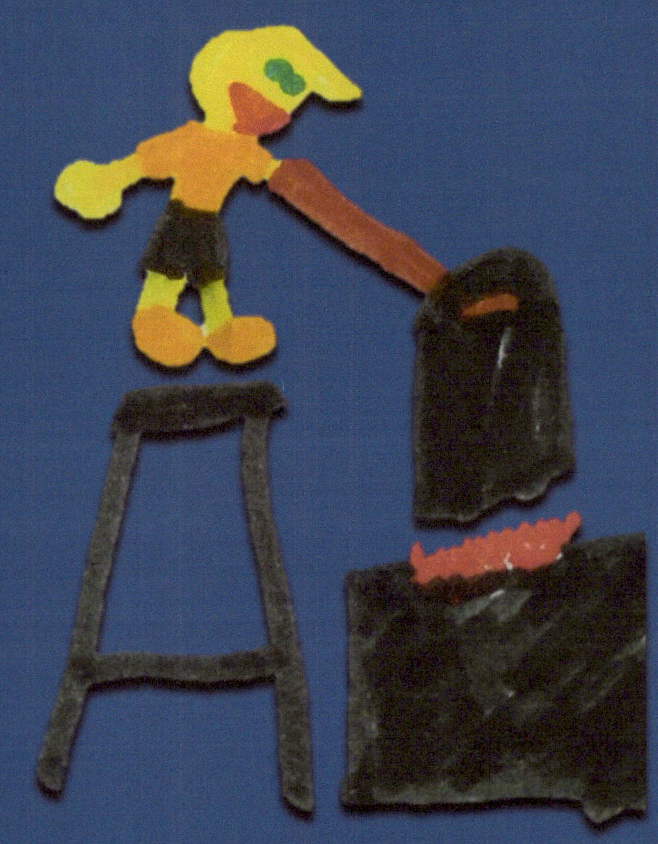

Here's a meal for you to try that might throw you for a loop.

It's a warm and sometimes spicy Moroccan chickpea soup.

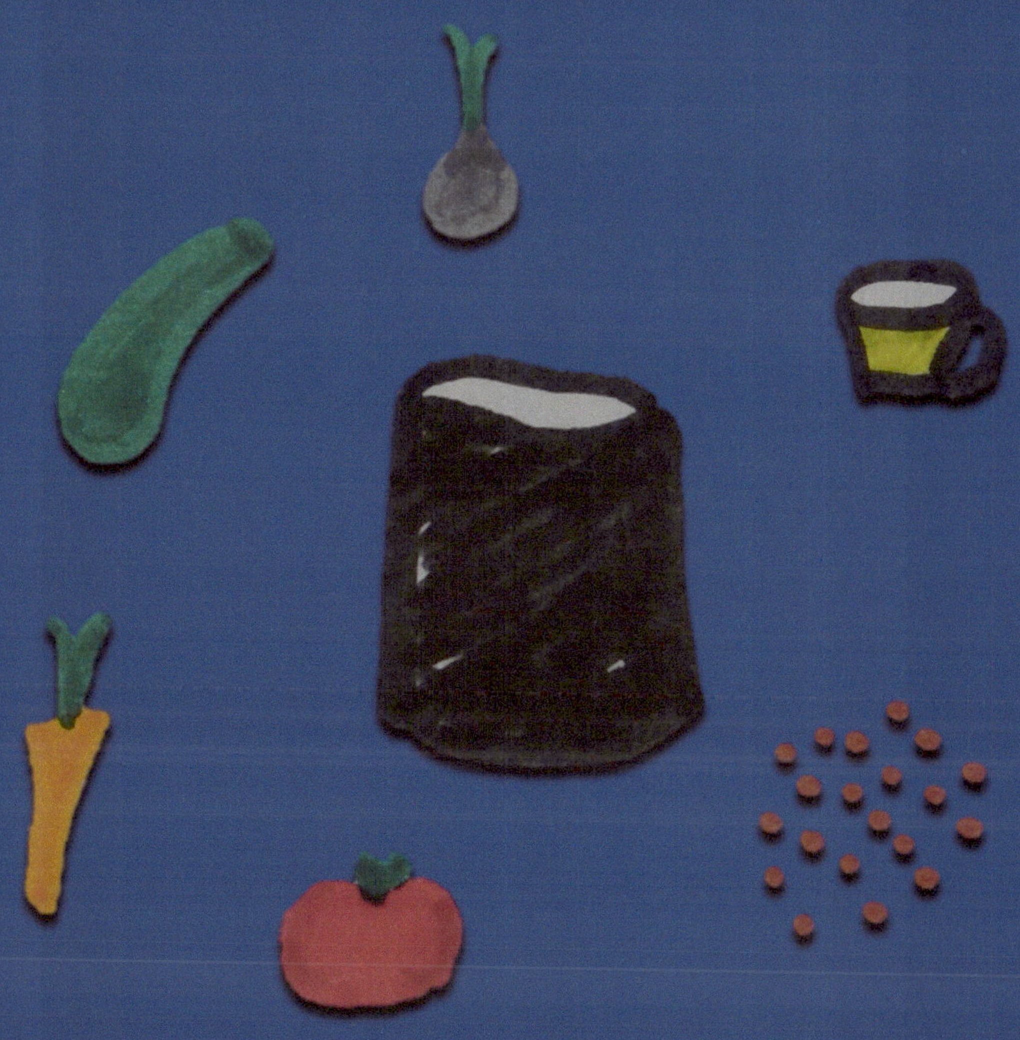

Vegetable broth makes up the base and chickpeas by the bunch.

Add in a ton of vegetables and this is one healthy lunch.

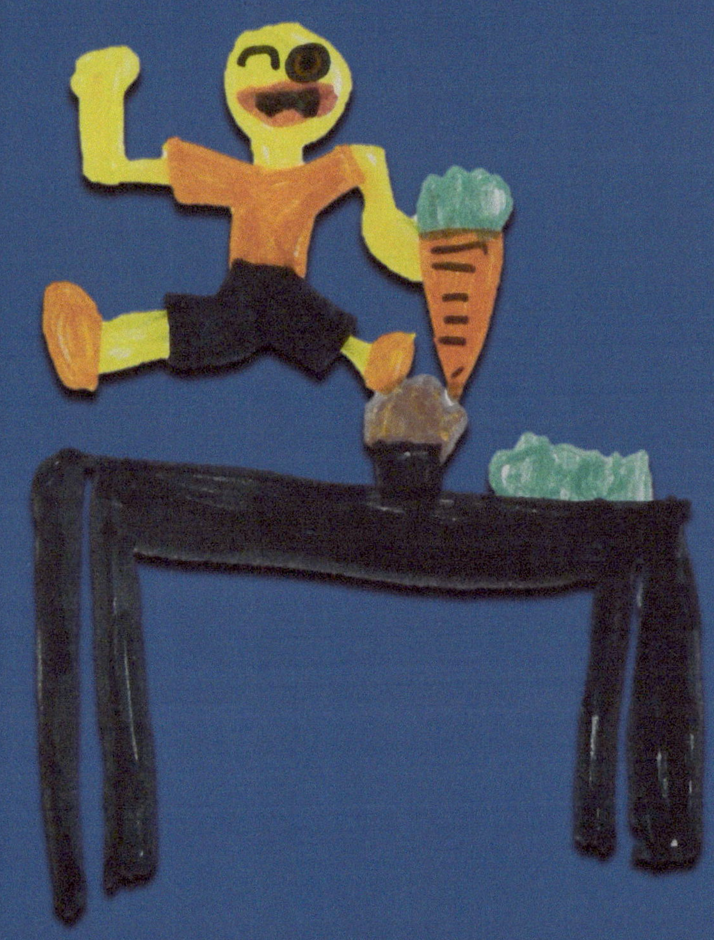

This one may not be a meal, but I eat hummus with a spoon.

I sometimes use a carrot when we're eating lunch at noon.

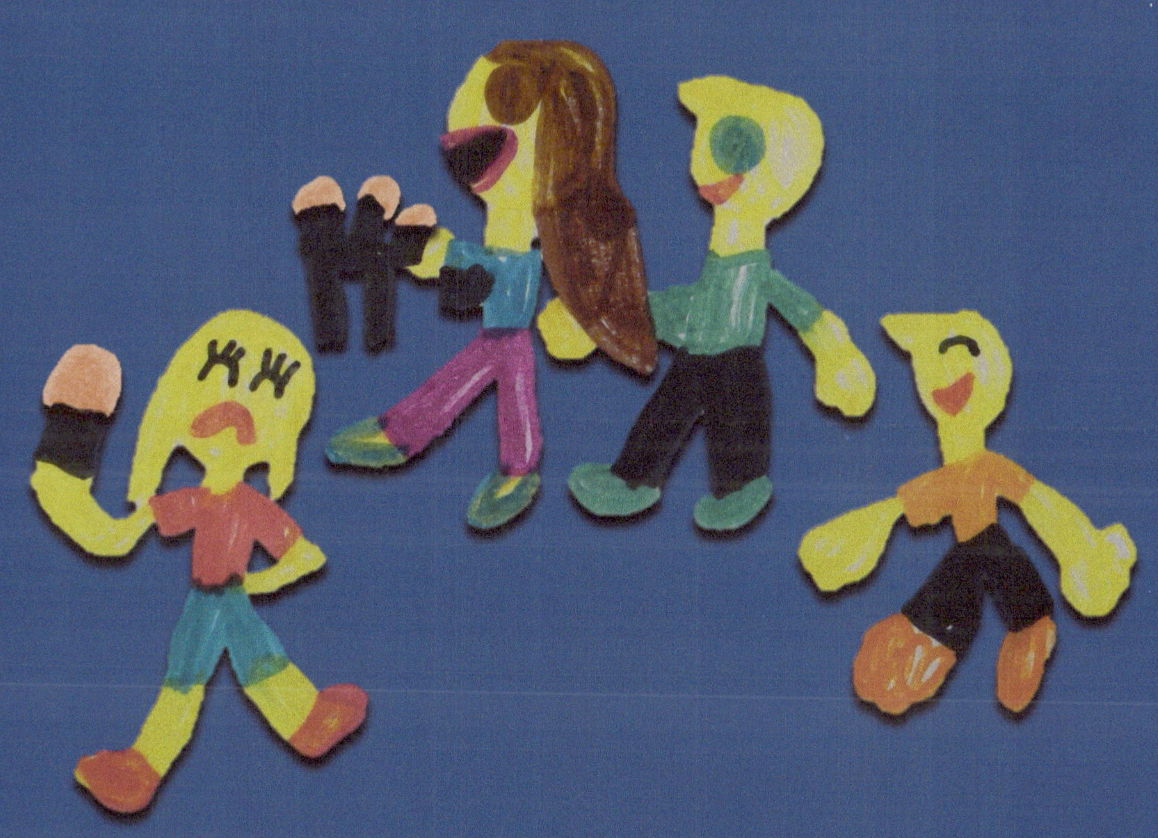

My mom and dad love hummus too, my sister's not a fan.

It's one of my favorite options when I'm hungry without a plan.

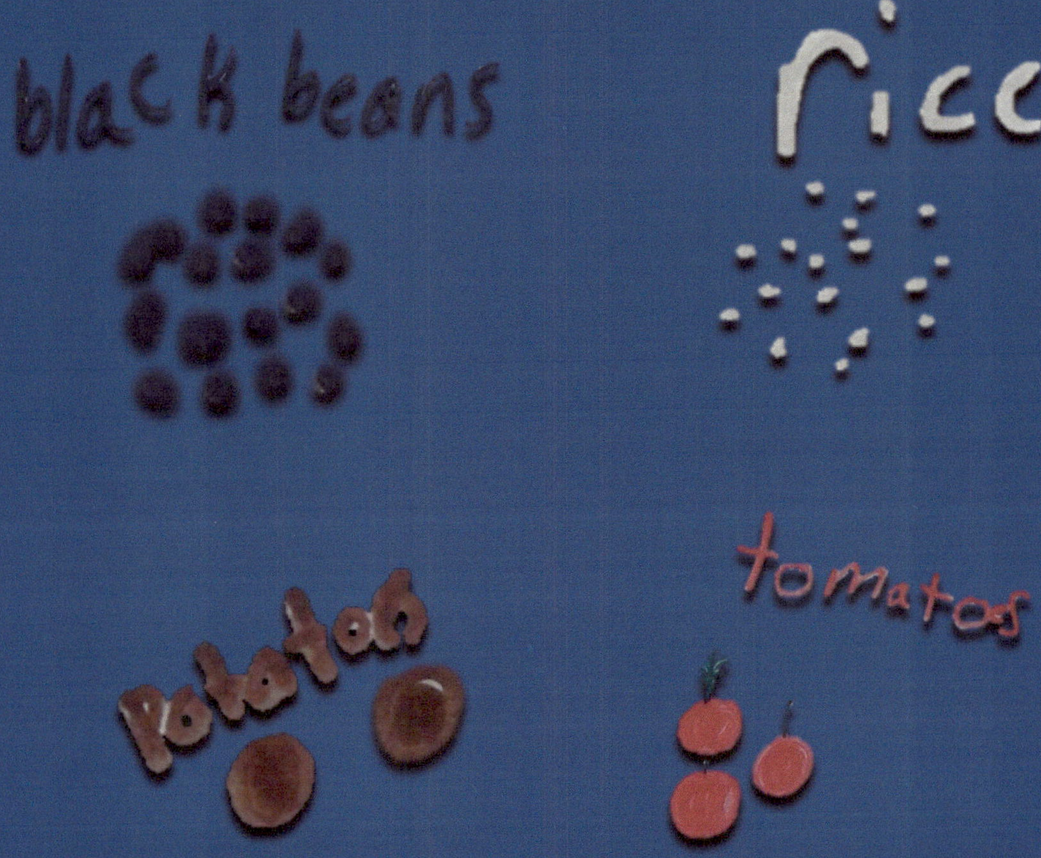

This next one fills me up and is full of rice and beans.

I call it a burrito bowl and it's served with a side of greens.

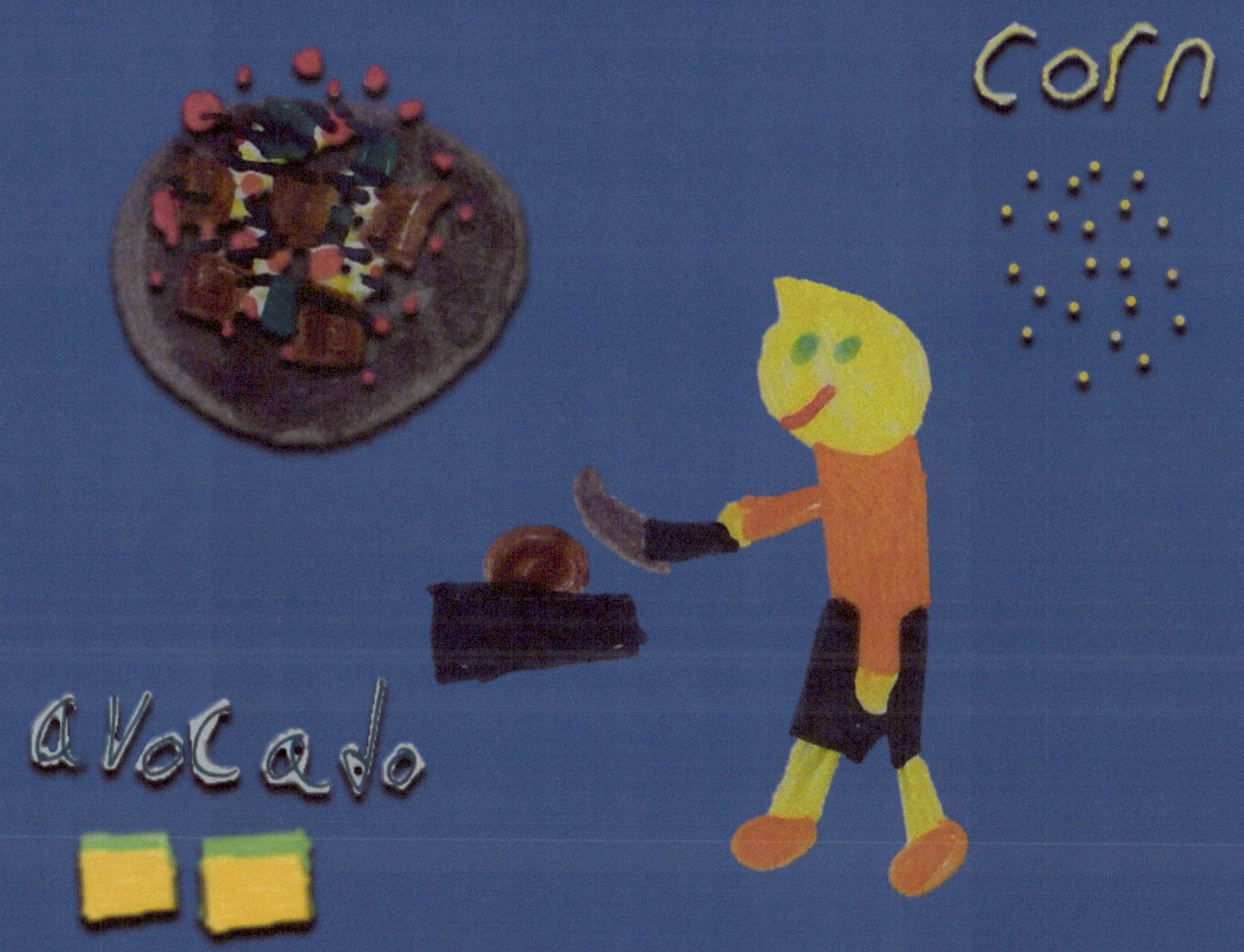

Add in some potatoes and vegan nacho cheese.

Don't forget the corn and avocado, if you please.

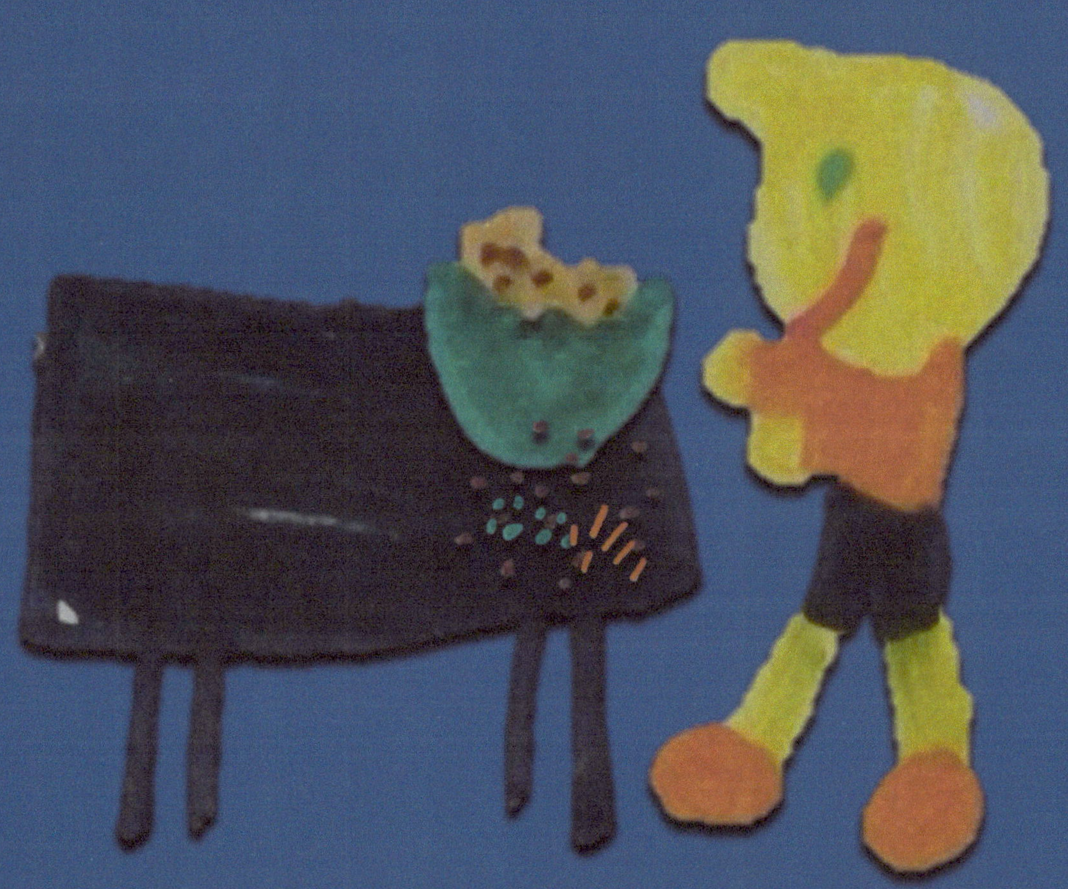

If I really want some protein, I make tofu lettuce wraps.

They can get a little messy, but I eat up all the scraps.

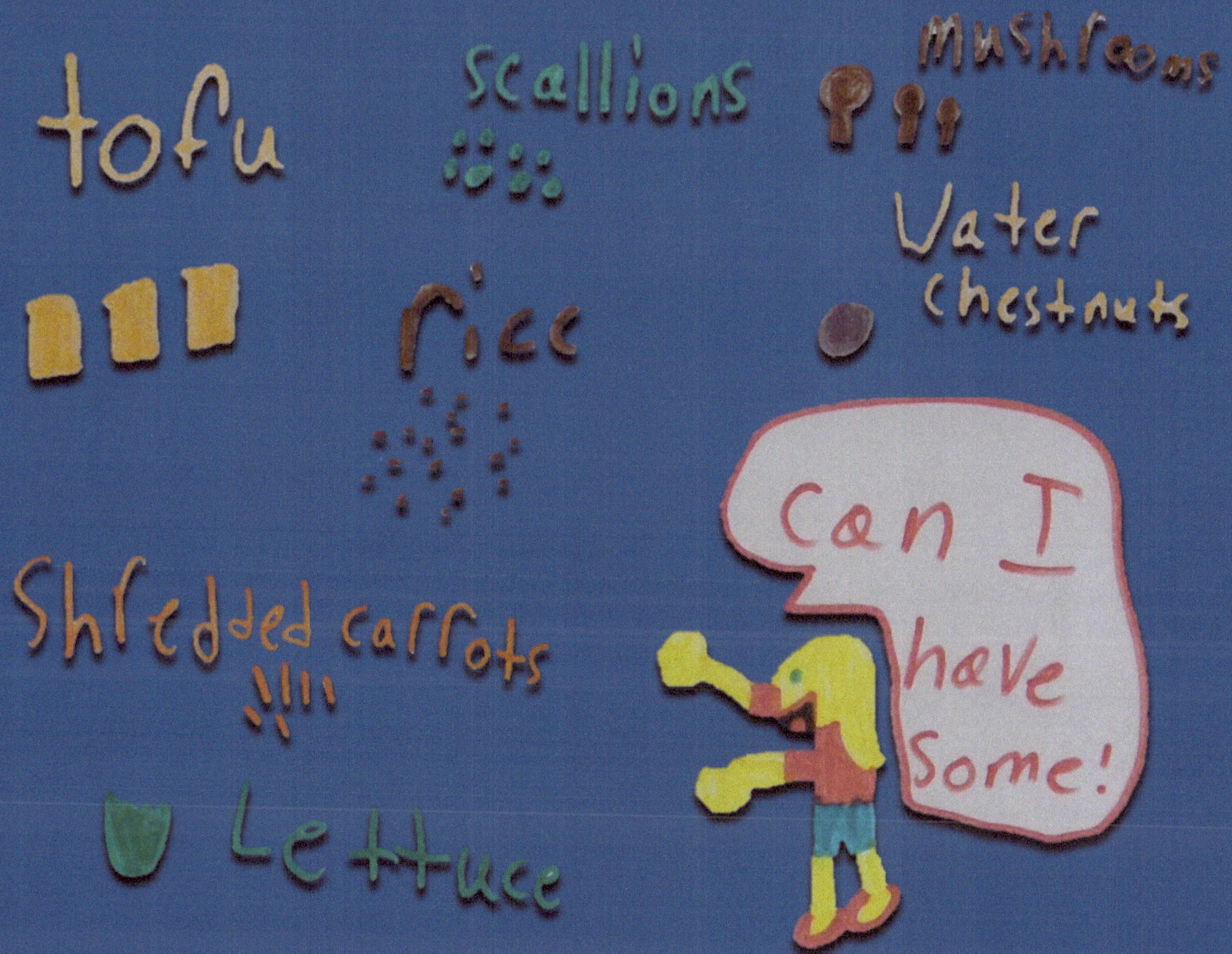

Water chestnuts, carrots, mushrooms, rice and yummy sauce.

My sister would eat this everyday if she was the boss.

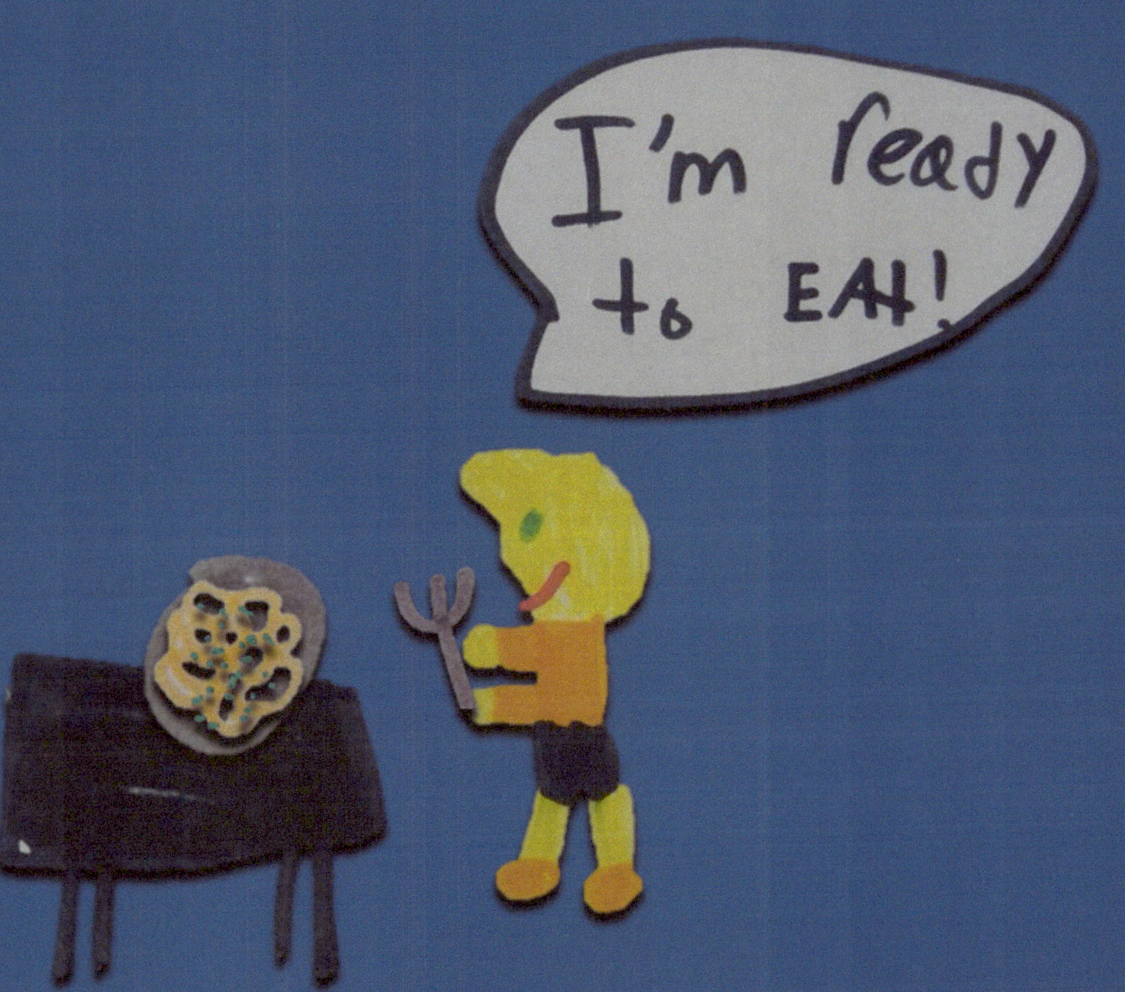

Me, I'd go with pad thai, though its really tough to say.

I think this is the meal I would choose to eat each and everyday.

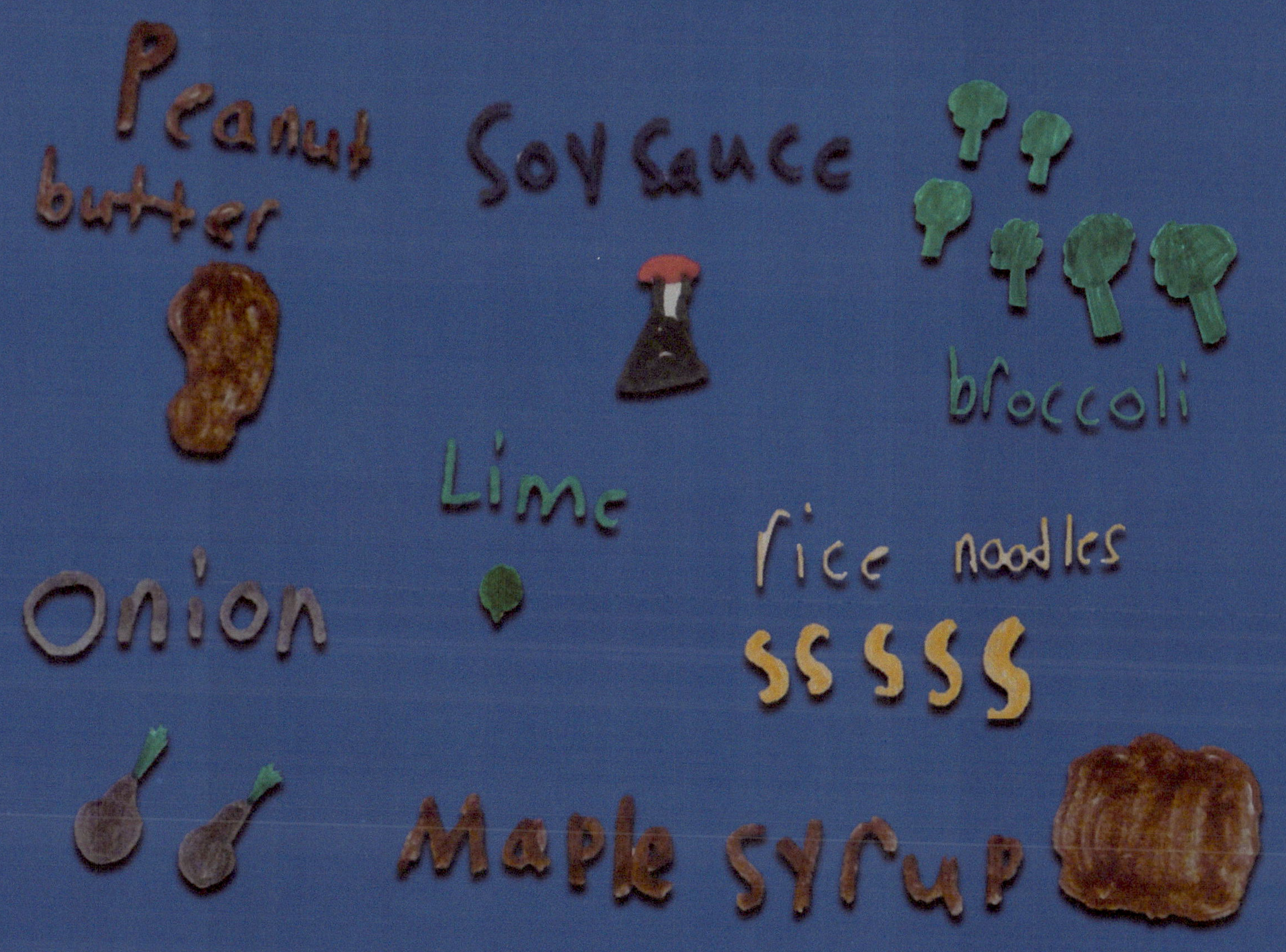

Peanut butter, broccoli, onions, soy sauce, lime, and maple syrup.

On top of rice noodles, it's amazing how good these stirrup.

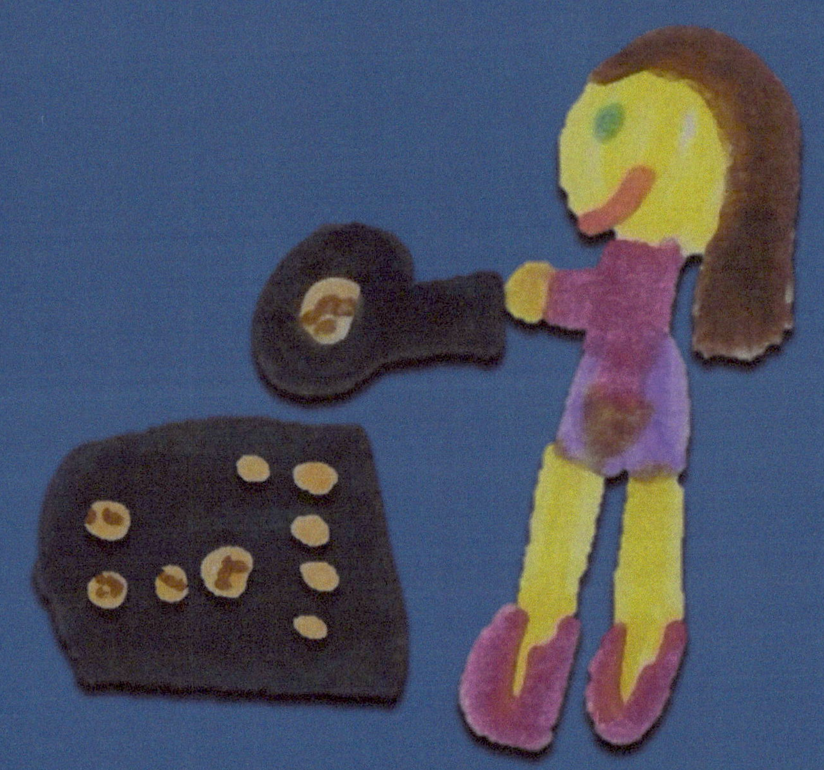

I've saved the best for last; the freshest homemade pancakes.

To get these on the table, I'd do whatever it takes.

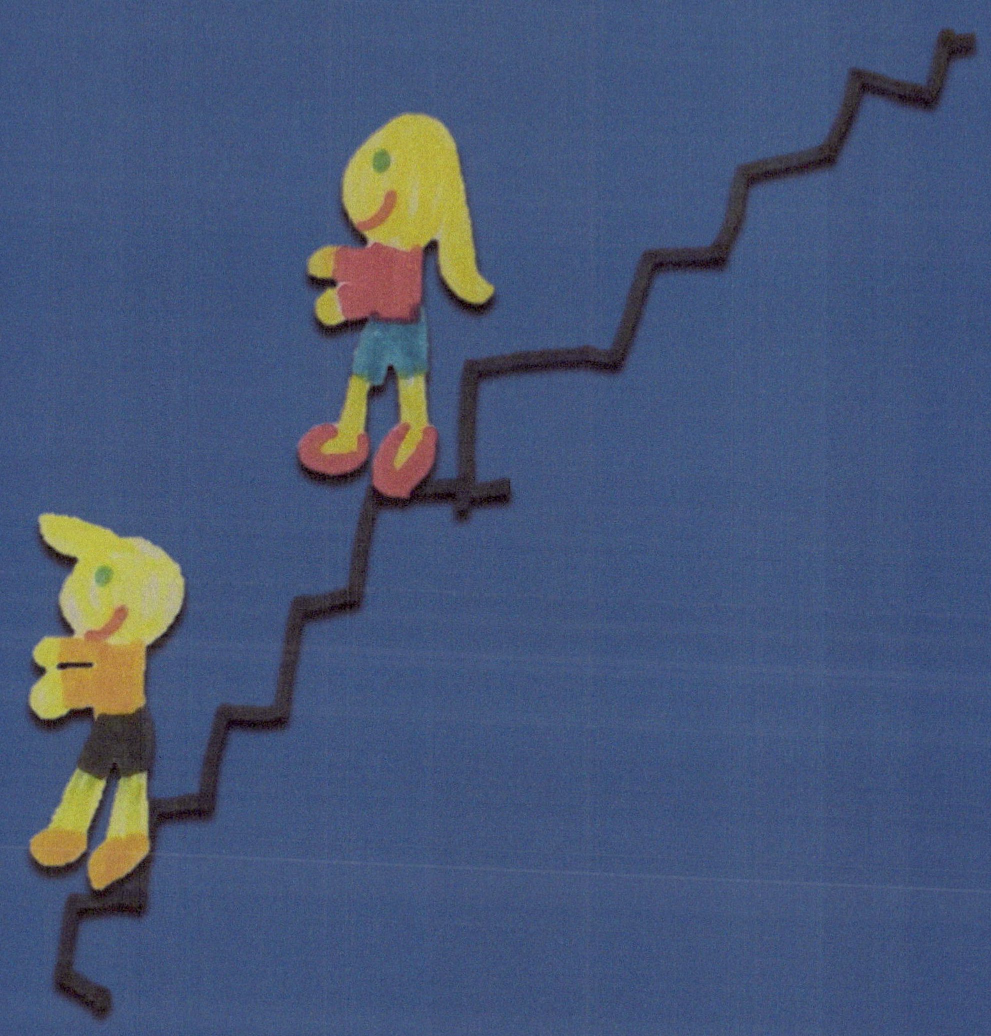

I sprint down to the kitchen like a tornado without warning.

I feel so warm and cozy at home with these on Saturday morning.

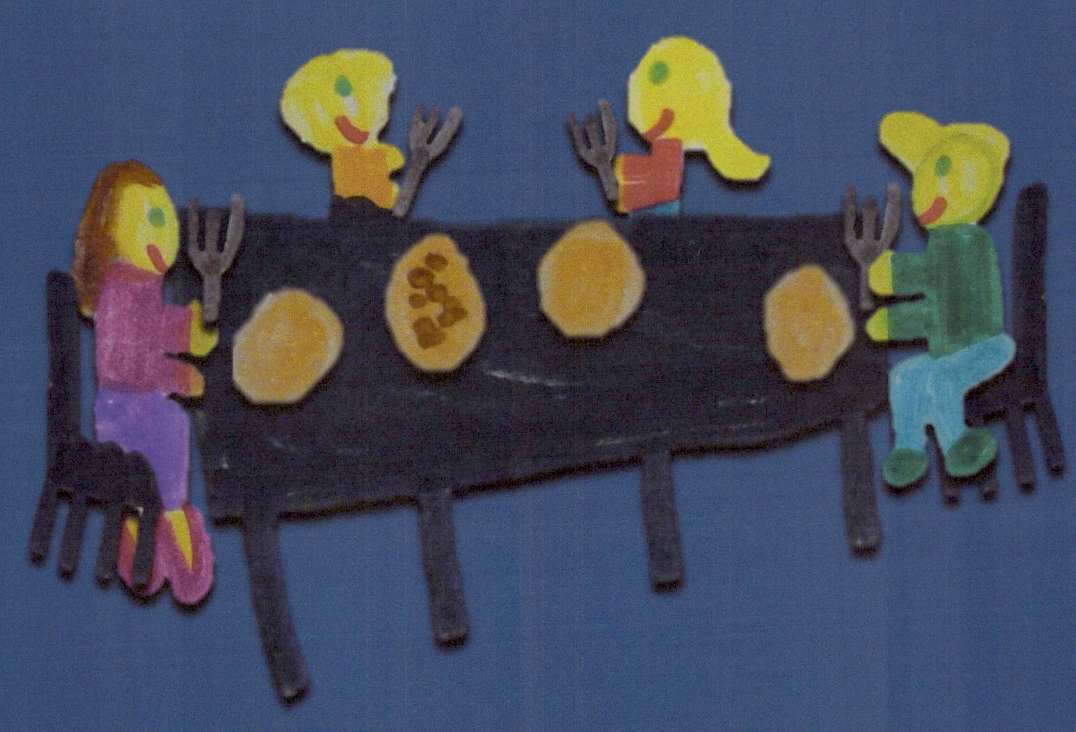

If you want to learn more about food and how it makes me feel,

come sit at my table and join me for a meal.

Resources for Parents:

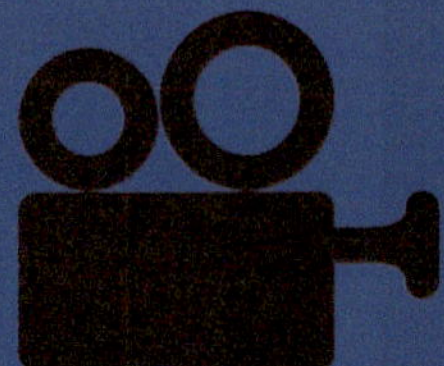

RECOMMENDED DOCUMENTARIES

*Forks Over Knives *What the Health *Vegucated *Cowspiracy *Food Choices
*Engine 2 Rescue *Before the Flood *The Game Changers *PlantPure Nation

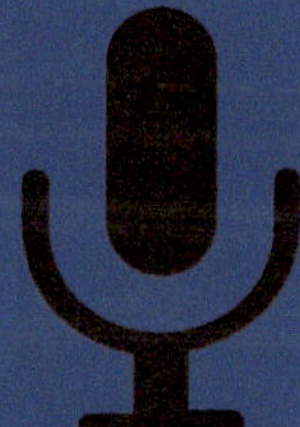

RECOMMENDED PODCASTS

*Stories of Self-Healing with Nurse Kristin *Jami Dulaney MD Plant Based
Wellness *Colleen Patrick-Goudreau: Food For Thought *The Exam Room:
Physicians Committee for Responsible Medicine

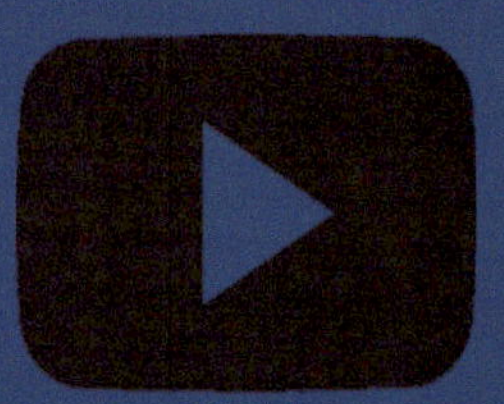

RECOMMENDED YOUTUBE CHANNELS/VIDEOS

*High Carb Hannah *Ellen Fisher *Best Speech You Will Ever Hear – Gary Yourofsky

<u>**Visit our website for more information:**</u>

Plantbasedpossibilities.com

"I give you every seed-bearing plant on the face of the whole earth and every tree that has fruit with seed in it. They will be yours for food. And to all the beasts of the earth and all the birds in the sky and all the creatures that move along the ground—everything that has the breath of life in it—I give every green plant for food." — Genesis 1:29-30

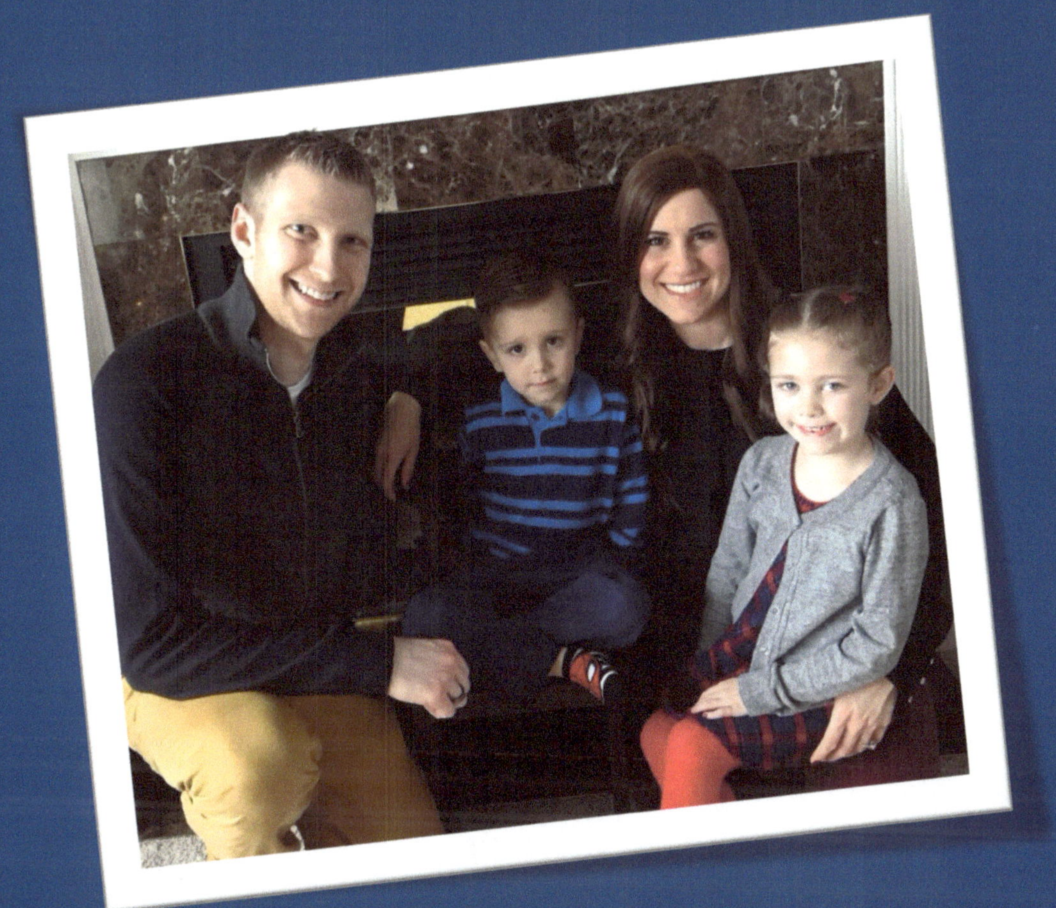

Hi there! We're the Greger Family and we have been living a plant-based lifestyle since May of 2017. Our journey started way before that though, as it has been a slow progression of finding health, energy, and what works for us and our two children. We have learned a lot along our way to becoming a plant-based family and want to share our experience and hopefully encourage others to join this movement. We know this is what's best for us, our planet, and our fellow creatures that roam the earth.